Uric Acid Optimization Diet

Eating for Weight Loss, Blood Sugar Control, and Vitality

By

Virgie W. Miller

Copyright

Introduction

Welcome to the amazing world of the "Uric Acid Optimization Diet: Eating for Weight Loss, Blood Sugar Control, and Vitality," a paradigm-shifting manual that not only promises a radical change in your eating habits but also in your general health and well-being. This thorough book stands out as a beacon of scientific integrity and holistic vitality in an era of many diet fads and health trends. Prepare to set off on a voyage that goes beyond the ordinary as we investigate the many dimensions of improving health through the management of uric acid.

In our investigation, uric acid—often ignored in traditional health discourse—takes center stage. We cordially welcome you to explore this substance's subtleties in order to comprehend the crucial part it plays in maintaining your body's health. While people only identify uric acid with ailments like gout, our guide reveals its broad impact on a variety of health issues, including metabolism, inflammation, and even energy levels.

But this isn't just a scientific adventure; it's also a useful road map for anyone looking for observable outcomes. Our goal is to arm you with the information and resources you need to control your blood sugar levels as well as lose excess weight. We combine the fields of weight loss, metabolic stability, and vitality improvement on this path.

This thorough manual's pages will reveal the following:

Scientific Groundwork: We debunk the myths around uric acid science so that you can fully appreciate its importance to your health. Understanding the science will enable you to choose your diet with greater knowledge.

Practical Strategies: Equipped with knowledge, we offer you practical advice on how to successfully implement the uric acid optimization diet into your everyday routine. We are aware that sustainable choices, rather than extreme constraints, are the key to long-lasting change.

Culinary delights include Bid adieu to boring, uninspired diet food. Our cookbook offers a tempting selection of dishes that suit a range of preferences and tastes. You'll discover a variety of culinary delights that will leave you happy and enthusiastic about your newfound nutritional route, from tasty breakfast alternatives to full, satisfying feasts.

Rejuvenated Vitality: You should anticipate a spectacular resurgence of vitality and well-being as you set off on your trip. More than merely a dietary shift, lowering your uric acid levels will help you feel more alive, energized, and rejuvenated.

So, are you ready to start moving in the direction of a happier, healthier self? This is more than simply a book; it is your compass for navigating the treacherous landscape of contemporary nutrition and succeeding in your struggle for a healthier life. Your passport to a happier, healthier future where you recover control over your health and vigor is the "Uric Acid Optimization Diet." Welcome to this life-changing trip; your future is waiting.

Chapter 1

The Science of Uric Acid

What You Need to Know About Uric Acid

Although frequently overshadowed by more widely discussed health indicators like blood pressure or cholesterol, uric acid is an essential part of our bodies' biochemistry. Knowing what it is and how it affects our well-being is crucial for keeping a balanced and successful life because it plays a vital part in our health.

Let's first define what uric acid is. It is a naturally occurring waste product created when the body breaks down purines, which are nutrients produced by our cells and present in some diets. Usual uric acid excretion from the body occurs through urine after dissolving in the blood, passing through the kidneys, and finally leaving the body.

The exciting aspect is now: why is uric acid important? High uric acid levels can have negative health effects even when they serve some necessary purposes. Gout is the most well-known disorder linked to high uric acid. When uric acid crystals gather in the joints, gout develops as a form of arthritis, resulting in excruciating pain and swelling. So that's why if you've ever heard someone discuss gout about uric acid.

However, gout isn't the only issue. Other health issues have also been connected to high uric acid levels. There is mounting evidence, for instance, that excess uric acid may be a factor in hypertension (high blood pressure), kidney stones, and even metabolic syndrome, which includes obesity, insulin resistance, and abnormal lipid profiles.

It's interesting to note that uric acid isn't the only bad guy in this health tale. Additionally, it functions in our blood as an antioxidant, aiding in the scavenging of dangerous free radicals. The complexity of uric acid's dual nature in our bodies is highlighted by this.

So what can you do to maintain healthy uric acid levels? Dietary habits are important. Levels of uric acid can be increased by purine-rich foods such as organ meats, some types of shellfish, and some alcoholic beverages. On the other hand, keeping uric acid levels in check can be achieved by eating a balanced diet, drinking plenty of water, and avoiding drinking too much alcohol.

Exercise regularly is also essential. Exercise can enhance insulin sensitivity, lower uric acid levels, and help with weight management. Furthermore, if you have a history of gout or persistently high uric acid levels, your doctor may recommend drugs to help you properly control it.

In essence, comprehending uric acid is comprehending a portion of the complex biochemistry of your body. Maintaining this balance is important for your general health. You can achieve balance in your uric acid levels, which will ultimately improve your health, by keeping an eye on your diet, remaining active, and seeking medical advice as required.

The Relationship Between Blood sugar, Weight ad Uric Acid

Let's explore the fascinating interactions between uric acid, weight, and blood sugar, a powerful trio that has a big impact on our health and well-being.

Our cells' main source of energy is blood sugar or glucose. In order to keep it within a very small range, it is strictly regulated in our bodies. Our bodies convert carbs into glucose during digestion, which raises our blood sugar levels. In reaction, the pancreas secretes the hormone insulin, which aids in bringing glucose into our cells for use as fuel or storage.

Let's now include weight in the calculation. Our body weight, particularly when it is excessive, can significantly affect how well our blood sugar is regulated. In particular, obesity and insulin resistance are tightly related. This means that when you are overweight, your cells are less sensitive to the signals from insulin. As a result, more insulin is needed to maintain normal blood sugar levels.

Uric acid now enters the picture. Obesity and high uric acid levels have been linked. Insulin resistance can result from uric acid buildup in the body. It is thought to disrupt the insulin signaling pathways, which makes it more difficult for glucose to enter cells efficiently. Consequently, the blood sugar levels rise.

Furthermore, the condition known as metabolic syndrome is frequently linked to excess weight, particularly in the abdominal region. A number of risk factors, including high blood pressure, diabetes, aberrant lipid profiles, and, intriguingly, high uric acid levels, are associated with this syndrome. Similar to a domino effect, one problem can lead to or aggravate another.

Don't forget about gout, the excruciating joint condition associated with excessive uric acid. Gout is more common in people who have metabolic syndrome and obesity, both of which are linked to high blood sugar levels. This shows that various components interact in a complicated web.

It's important to stress that this relationship is multifaceted though. It resembles a complex dance where one part affects the others. For instance, managing weight can have a good effect on blood sugar regulation. Losing extra weight frequently results in increased insulin sensitivity and better blood sugar control.

What can we learn from this complex connection, then? It just goes to show how crucial a comprehensive approach to health is. A healthy lifestyle that incorporates a balanced diet, regular exercise, and weight control can support the maintenance of normal blood sugar levels and may also have a good impact on uric acid. To advance general well-being, this dynamic three must work toward harmony.

Chapter 2

Checking Your Levels of Uric Acid

Managing your health and avoiding potential problems like gout, high blood pressure, and kidney stones requires an understanding of your uric acid levels. We'll now explore how to measure your uric acid levels and what the results can indicate for your health.

Blood test, First A blood test is the main technique for determining uric acid levels. A little sample of blood is simply drawn from a vein in your arm during this simple procedure by a medical professional. The sample is subsequently delivered to a lab for evaluation. Typically, the data are presented as milligrams per deciliter (mg/dL) values.

Normal Range In general: the normal range for uric acid levels is between 2.4 and 6.0 mg/dL for women and 3.4 to 7.0 mg/dL for males, however, it can vary significantly between laboratories. Remember that what is deemed "normal" might change depending on things like age, sex, and personal health.

Interpreting Results: Knowing the numbers alone won't help you understand your uric acid results. Hyperuricemia, or elevated uric acid levels, can be a sign of several illnesses, such as gout, kidney disease, metabolic syndrome, or even a diet high in purines. On the other hand, abnormally low uric acid levels can potentially indicate some medical conditions.

Clinical Evaluation: The findings of your uric acid test must be interpreted in light of your medical history, way of life, and any symptoms you may be feeling. For instance, signs like joint discomfort along with high uric acid levels may point to gout.

Consulting a Medical Professional: It's critical to speak with a healthcare professional if your uric acid levels are over normal or if you have any worries about your health. They can advise you, carry out additional tests if necessary, and collaborate with you to create an individual plan for managing your uric acid levels and general health.

Lifestyle adjustments: Your healthcare professional could suggest lifestyle adjustments based on your uric acid levels and particular medical concerns. This can entail dietary changes, more water, managing weight, or taking uric acid-lowering medicines.

Regular inspection: It is frequently required to monitor your uric acid levels over time, particularly if you have a history of high uric acid levels or have been diagnosed with a disorder like gout. Blood tests performed regularly can be used to monitor your development and the success of any interventions.

Measuring your uric acid levels is a useful tool for learning about your health. The context in which the statistics appear on the lab report is just as important as the numbers themselves. Working together with your doctor and taking a proactive approach to con Managing trolling your uric acid levels will help you take charge of your health and lower your chance of developing related conditions.

Charting Your Path to Wellness: Setting Your Health Goals

Setting definite, doable goals is the first step in starting along the path to greater health. Your health goals act as compass points to lead you through the complex landscape of well-being. In order to live a happier, healthier life, let's discuss how to set, prioritize, and work toward these goals.

Self-reflection: First Start by carefully examining your present state of health and way of life. What are the drawbacks you face? Which elements of your health need to be improved? Do you want to target any particular health issues or conditions? The first step in developing a roadmap for your health journey is recognizing where you are.

Specify Your Goals: It's time to define your health objectives after you've evaluated your current position. These objectives must be SMART, specified, measurable, achievable, relevant, and time-limited. For instance, set a specific goal like "reduce 10 pounds in the next three months through a balanced diet and frequent exercise," as opposed to a general one like "lose weight."

Prioritize Your Objectives: It's important to prioritize your health goals even if you have multiple ones in mind. Think about the objectives that are most important to you or that will have the biggest impact on your general wellbeing. You can direct your attention and resources where they will have the biggest impact by using prioritization.

Break It Down: Lofty objectives might occasionally feel daunting. Divide them into smaller, easier-to-handle steps. If your objective is to run a marathon, for instance, start by planning to complete a 5K race in the coming months. These small victories along the way keep you inspired and give you a sense of progress.

Seek Advice from a Professional: Consulting a doctor, nutritionist, or fitness trainer can offer helpful insights and advice that are catered to your particular requirements and goals. They can aid in the development of a unique plan and the tracking of your advancement.

Have Reasonable Expectations: Though lofty objectives are admirable, they should also be attainable. Unfounded hopes can cause annoyance and disappointment. Be realistic about what you can accomplish given your circumstances and time constraints.

Create a Support System: Tell your loved ones about your health objectives so they can support you and hold you accountable. Think about participating in support groups or looking for people who have similar goals to yourself. A strong motivator can be having a network of supporters.

Monitor Your Progress: Maintaining focus requires keeping track of your progress. Use wearable technology, a fitness app, or a journal to keep track of your accomplishments. By regularly assessing your results, you can change your tactics as necessary.

Remain adaptable: Since life is erratic, every path will inevitably include obstacles. View setbacks as opportunities to learn and modify your strategy rather than failures. For long-term success, flexibility and adaptation are essential.

Rejoice in Your Successes: Celebrate your accomplishments, no matter how minor they may seem. Recognizing your successes helps you stay motivated and committed to your health goals.

Setting your health objectives is a significant act of self-care and self-improvement, to sum up. It involves imagining your healthiest self and taking action to achieve that vision. You may start down a path to better health and a happier, healthier life if you have clear goals, a strong network of allies, and a resilient mindset.

Chapter 3

Crafting Your Uric Acid-Friendly Eating Plan

Foods that Lower Uric Acid Levels

A balanced diet can be your ally if you're trying to keep your uric acid levels in check or lower your chances of developing illnesses like gout. It has been demonstrated that a few foods can reduce uric acid levels and the accompanying health hazards. Let's look at some of the items you can eat to help reduce your uric acid intake.

Cherries: The ability of cherries to lower uric acid levels has attracted interest, especially tart cherries. They contain substances that might aid in reducing inflammation and uric acid generation.

Berries: In addition to being delicious, berries like strawberries, blueberries, and blackberries are also high in antioxidants. These antioxidants may reduce inflammation and help to reduce uric acid levels.

Apples: Apples are renowned for their fiber content, which can indirectly affect uric acid levels and assist control of blood sugar levels. They make for an easy and nutritious snack option.

Citrus fruits like oranges, lemons, and grapefruits are just a few that are excellent sources of vitamin C. Increasing your intake of citrus fruits can be advantageous because vitamin C has been linked to lower uric acid levels.

Low-Fat Dairy: In addition to being calcium-rich, low-fat dairy products like skim milk and yogurt may also help decrease uric acid levels. They seem to have a gout-prevention effect.

Fiber is abundant in whole grains. Examples of whole grains are brown rice, whole wheat, and oats. Fiber may indirectly influence the metabolism of uric acid by assisting in the control of insulin and blood sugar levels.

Leafy Greens: Kale and spinach are two examples of dark, leafy greens that are rich in minerals and antioxidants. They have low quantities of purines, which can result in higher levels of uric acid.

Nuts: Almonds in particular can be a wise snack option for uric acid management. They can serve as a tasty, healthful alternative to commercial food and are low in purines.

Fatty Fish: Omega-3 fatty acids are abundant in fatty fish including salmon, mackerel, and trout. The anti-inflammatory effects of omega-3 fatty acids may assist in reducing uric acid levels.

Water: Despite not being a food, drinking plenty of water is essential for uric acid regulation. To assist your kidneys in removing extra uric acid from your body, drink plenty of water.

Coffee: Here is some good news for coffee drinkers. Lower uric acid levels have been associated with moderate coffee drinking. Just be cautious of high-fat creamers or additional sweets.

Tofu: For those worried about their uric acid levels, tofu, a plant-based source of protein, is a good substitute for animal proteins because it normally contains fewer purines.

Although certain meals may be advantageous, it's important to keep a well-balanced diet and take your overall nutritional requirements into account. Consult a medical expert or qualified dietitian if you have specific questions about uric acid levels or gout. They can offer individualized dietary advice that is catered to your particular health profile.

Building Balanced Meals

Meal plans that aim to reduce uric acid levels must carefully evaluate the right foods and their appropriate ratios. Let's explore the key ingredients for creating meals that promote uric acid control and general wellness.

Begin with a balanced protein diet: Start your meal with a protein source because controlling uric acid levels depends on it. Excellent choices for lean foods include poultry, fish, tofu, lentils, and beans. Give your protein around a quarter of your dish.

Boost the Vegetable Quotient: The optimization of uric acid is significantly influenced by vegetables. They are naturally low in purines, which can cause increased uric acid levels, and they offer vital minerals and fiber. Aim to have a variety of colorful veggies, such as broccoli, peppers, and leafy greens, on at least half of your plate.

Include carbohydrates that are friendly to uric acid: Include uric acid-friendly complex carbs in your diet. Brown rice, quinoa, and whole wheat pasta are all great examples of whole grains. These carbohydrates give you long-lasting energy without having a big effect on your uric acid. They ought to fill around half of your plate.

Accept Healthy Fats: Don't be afraid of good fats. They can enhance a meal that is uric acid-optimized and is necessary for overall wellness. Your diet becomes richer as a result of sources like avocados, almonds, seeds, and olive oil. Put fats on about a quarter of your plate.

Fiber's Crucial Function: Fiber, which is abundant in vegetables, legumes, and whole grains, is a friend in the management of uric acid. It controls blood sugar levels and supports intestinal health. Give high-fiber foods like whole grains and lentils a top priority.

Portion Control Considerations: To avoid overeating, keep portion control. You may receive a balance of nutrients with proper portion control without overdosing your body. Pay attention to your body's signals and stop eating once you're full.

Keep Hydrated: Water intake must be adequate for uric acid regulation. Water helps your body wash out extra uric acid. Include water with your meal, and don't forget to keep drinking water throughout the day to maintain optimum hydration.

Reduce the intake of sugar and processed foods: Limit your intake of meals and beverages with lots of processed and added sugars. These can affect uric acid levels and cause weight gain. To reduce uric acid, eat only whole, minimally processed foods.

Mindfulness in Eating: To appreciate each bite and feel connected to your meal, try mindful eating. It supports the regulation of uric acid by making it easier for you to know when you're full and preventing overeating. Make a distraction-free, concentrated dining space.

Dietary preferences and limitations: Your uric acid-optimized meals should be modified to satisfy any dietary preferences or requirements you may have. Make sure your meals reflect your dietary preferences while still placing a high priority on uric acid management, regardless of whether you practice a vegetarian, vegan, or gluten-free diet.

Creating meals that are uric acid optimized is a personalized strategy for keeping your health. Adapt your meals to your nutritional needs, degree of activity, and uric acid management objectives. You can establish the groundwork for uric acid optimization and general health by planning meals that combine a variety of nutrients and food types.

Meal Timing and Portion Control

The time of your meals and portion control are crucial in the effort to reduce your uric acid levels. You can keep your uric acid levels more consistent throughout the day by using these methods. Let's examine the importance of portion control and meal timing for uric acid optimization.

Regular Meal Timing: Setting up a regular eating plan can help with uric acid management. Try to eat at about the same time every day. This consistency aids in controlling the generation and excretion of uric acid as well as other metabolic processes in your body.

Prevent Skipping Meals: Missing meals can cause unstable blood sugar levels, especially at breakfast. Fluctuations in blood sugar might affect insulin sensitivity and, as a result, uric acid levels. Try to consume well-balanced meals on a regular basis.

Portion Management: In order to avoid overeating, which can lead to weight gain and higher uric acid levels, portion control is crucial. When serving meals, use smaller plates and pay attention to portion proportions. Pay attention to your hunger signals so you can stop eating when you're full.

Balanced Snacking: Pick uric acid-friendly foods if you must snack in between meals. Choose healthy snacks like low-fat yogurt, fresh fruit, or a few nuts to keep your energy levels stable without significantly raising your uric acid levels.

Drink Water Throughout the Day: Optimizing uric acid requires maintaining hydration. Regularly sip water throughout the day to help your kidneys remove extra uric acid from your body and improve renal function.

Mindful Eating: Make an effort to eat mindfully when you eat. Take your time, enjoy every bite, and focus on the tastes and textures of your meal. This strategy not only improves your dining experience but also teaches you to detect fullness and reduce overeating.

Avoid eating after midnight: Avoid eating large, fatty meals right before night. Eating after midnight may affect sleep patterns and raise uric acid levels. At least a few hours before retiring for the night, choose lighter, more balanced dinners.

Make a plan: Making a plan for your meals and snacks might help you choose healthier options. In order to avoid impulsive, less nutrient-dense choices, prepare meals that are uric acid-optimized and keep healthy snacks on hand.

Think About Fasting: Some people find that fasting intermittently is effective at controlling their uric acid levels. Fasting should be carried out under the supervision of a medical practitioner, though, as it may not be appropriate for everyone.

Watch Your Body's Reaction: Pay attention to how your body reacts to the size and timing of meals. Keep an eye out for variations in your uric acid levels as well as symptoms like gout attacks. You can use this information to help you improve your food planning.

A proactive strategy for uric acid optimization is to include meal timing and portion control in your daily diet. These practices help regulate blood sugar more effectively, which can help keep uric acid levels steady and lower the risk of related health problems. For the best uric acid control, adapt these tactics to your particular requirements and preferences.

Strategies for Dining Out

When eating out, maintaining uric acid optimization doesn't have to be difficult. You can enjoy eating at restaurants while making decisions that support your uric acid management objectives by using the correct tactics. Let's look at how to negotiate eating out while controlling your uric acid levels.

Examine the Menu Ahead of Time: A lot of restaurants offer their menus online. Utilize this by looking over the menu before you go. Choose uric acid-friendly foods like lean protein, salads, and recipes that are vegetable-based.

Select lean proteins: Choose lean proteins like grilled chicken, turkey, or fish when it comes to protein sources. Compared to red meats and organ meats, these choices have reduced purine content, which can help to cause increased uric acid levels.

Accept Plant-Based Alternatives: Salads, vegetable stir-fries, and bean-based dishes are examples of dishes that are plant-based. Purine levels are often lower in plant-based diets, which can also be pleasant and filling.

Be Conscious of Portions: Compared to what you would serve at home, restaurant portions are frequently bigger. Consider splitting an entree with a dining buddy or ordering a to-go container in advance to save half of your meal for later to help you control your intake.

Requesting Customizations: Never be afraid to request changes to your food. You can choose healthier options by asking for adjustments like steaming vegetables rather than frying them or dressing them on the side.

Keep an eye out for hidden sugars: Watch out for hidden added sugars in dressings and sauces. Consuming too much sugar can reduce insulin sensitivity and, in turn, hurt uric acid levels.

Select whole grains: Choose whole grains over refined grains if the restaurant has them. Energy from whole grains, such as brown rice or whole wheat pasta, is more steady and has less of an impact on uric acid levels.

Maintain Hydration: Do not forget to sip water before and during meals. Maintaining adequate hydration is essential for helping your kidneys process and remove uric acid from your body.

Limiting alcohol intake is important: Purines can be found in alcohol, particularly in beer and some cocktails, which may raise uric acid levels. If you prefer to drink, keep your intake under control or choose lower-purine options.

Engage in Mindful Eating: Eat slowly, chew food thoroughly, and pay attention to your body's hunger signals. Overindulgence can be avoided with mindful eating, which also supports uric acid control.

Think About Sharing Dessert: If you want to enjoy dessert, think about dividing it up among the people seated at your table. You can fulfill your sweet taste in this way without going overboard.

Plan for Success: If you anticipate eating out, make sure your other meals and snacks account for it. This can balance out your daily intake as a whole and lessen the negative effects of eating out on your uric acid levels.

Take pleasure in your dining experience: It's not just the food that matters when you eat out; it's also the experience. Make your dinner experience a complete one by concentrating on taking in the company of your dining companions and the atmosphere of the establishment.

Applying these techniques will let you enjoy eating out while being mindful of your uric acid intake. Keep in mind that flexibility and moderation are essential and that treating yourself once in a while is part of a well-rounded strategy for managing uric acid.

Chapter 4

Weight Loss and Uric Acid Control

Uric Acid and Weight Gain: The Connection

There is more to the connection between uric acid and weight growth than first appears. Let's investigate the relationship between these two elements and how they might affect one another.

Production of uric acid: When the body breaks down purines, which are substances present in some diets and also synthesized by our cells, uric acid is created as a natural waste product. When the body overproduces uric acid or when there are too many purines in the diet, elevated uric acid levels can result.

The Kidneys' Function: A balanced uric acid level is maintained in large part by having healthy kidneys. Extra uric acid is removed from the blood by filtering and is subsequently eliminated through urination. Whenever the kidneys aren't working at their best, uric acid can build up in the blood.

The Consequences of Weight Gain Numerous factors can cause weight growth, especially excessive body fat, to alter uric acid levels.

Insulin resistance, a condition in which cells don't react well to insulin, is intimately related to obesity. Because insulin resistance inhibits the kidneys' ability to excrete uric acid, increased uric acid levels can result.

Inflammation Adipose (fat) tissue is an active endocrine organ that secretes inflammatory chemicals in addition to serving as a passive energy storage facility. Production of uric acid may be encouraged by obesity-related chronic low-grade inflammation.

Diets Rich in Purine: Due to the high-calorie content of foods high in purines, obese people may consume diets that are higher in purines. This can result in more uric acid being produced.

Metabolic Syndrome: A key component of metabolic syndrome is weight gain, a collection of risk factors that also includes high blood pressure, aberrant lipid profiles, raised blood sugar, and, intriguingly, high uric acid levels. The effects of weight growth on uric acid are amplified by this syndrome, which acts as a magnifier.

Gout: A major risk factor for gout, a painful and inflammatory joint ailment, is having high uric acid levels. Obesity and excess weight are also linked to a higher chance of acquiring gout. These elements working together may cause gout attacks to occur more frequently.

Lifestyle factors include: When examining the link between uric acid and weight gain, lifestyle factors are crucial to take into account. Elevated uric acid levels and weight gain are frequently linked to sedentary behavior, poor dietary decisions, and excessive calorie consumption.

The Vicious Cycle: Increased uric acid can cause weight gain, and vice versa, weight gain can make uric acid problems worse. Each factor amplifies the effects of the others, creating a vicious cycle.

The significance of lifestyle changes: In many cases, controlling uric acid levels and avoiding weight gain go hand in hand. A balanced diet, regular exercise, maintaining a healthy weight, and avoiding an excessive amount of foods high in purines are all lifestyle changes that can help break the cycle and advance general well-being.

There are several ways in which uric acid and weight gain are related. Through a variety of mechanisms, both factors can affect one another and have an impact on general health. The significance of a holistic approach to health that addresses both uric acid management and weight control to achieve optimal well-being is highlighted by the recognition of this interplay.

Strategies for Healthy and Sustainable Weight Loss

Controlling uric acid levels requires achieving and maintaining a healthy weight. Here are some strategies for controlling uric acid levels while making long-term, healthy weight loss.

A balanced diet Concentrate on eating a balanced diet with a few items high in purines. Choose healthy grains over refined grains, including lots of veggies, and lean proteins like poultry and fish. Limit your consumption of high-purine shellfish, organ meats, and red meat.

Portion control: Consider the sizes of your servings. You may prevent overeating and control calorie intake by using smaller plates, measuring your meals, and paying attention to the recommended portion sizes.

Consistent Meals: Avoid missing meals and stick to your normal mealtimes. Your blood sugar levels can be stabilized by maintaining consistency in your dietary habits, which is advantageous for uric acid optimization.

Hydration: Make sure you're getting enough water throughout the day to stay hydrated. Maintaining proper water helps the kidneys remove extra uric acid.

Steer clear of sugary beverages: Reduce your intake of sugary beverages like fruit juices and soda. These may indirectly impact uric acid levels and contribute to weight gain.

Select Nutritious Snacks: Choose nutritious options like fruits, veggies, and unsalted almonds if you need a snack in between meals. Avoid snacks with lots of calories but few nutrients.

Mindful Consumption: By focusing on what you eat, enjoying every bite, and paying attention to your body's hunger cues, you can practice mindful eating. Avoid eating while distracted, such as when watching TV or using a computer.

Regular exercise is a must: Make regular exercise a part of your regimen. Strive to perform a variety of Exercise boosts insulin sensitivity and helps you lose weight, both of which are beneficial for lowering uric acid levels. Strive to perform a variety of aerobic strength-training workouts.

Gradual Alterations: Make sustainable, modest modifications to your eating and exercise routines. Extreme diets and strenuous exercise regimens can be hard to keep up over the long run and may not result in lasting weight loss.

Seek Support: Take into account collaborating with a doctor, licensed nutritionist, or weight reduction coach. They can advise you, keep track of your development, and make tailored suggestions depending on your particular requirements.

Track Your Progress: Keep tabs on your uric acid levels as well as the amount of weight you're losing.

You can stay on track and make modifications as necessary with regular monitoring.

Set realistic objectives: Set attainable weight-loss targets that complement your overall health goals. It is frequently more sustainable and healthy to aim for a weight loss of 1-2 pounds steadily and gradually each week as opposed to losing a lot of weight quickly.

Put Your Health Overall First: Maintaining optimal uric acid levels is important for overall health, not only for weight loss. Adopt a holistic strategy that incorporates a nutritious diet, regular exercise, and other lifestyle choices.

By incorporating these techniques into your daily routine, you can support uric acid optimization while working toward healthy and long-lasting weight loss.

Keep in mind that improving your health is a marathon, not a sprint and that consistency is the key to success over the long haul.

Including Exercise to Control Uric Acid

Exercise is a significant technique in the treatment of uric acid levels. Physical activity benefits in numerous ways:

Weight Management: Regular exercise aids in weight control, reducing the risk of obesity, a factor connected to high uric acid levels.

Improved Insulin Sensitivity: Exercise raises the body's sensitivity to insulin, which can lead to better blood sugar regulation and indirectly impact uric acid levels.

Enhanced Kidney Function: Physical exercise helps kidney health, assisting in the effective elimination of excess uric acid from the body.

Reduced Inflammation: Exercise has anti-inflammatory properties that can help decrease uric acid-related inflammation.

Joint Health: For patients with gout, exercise can maintain joint flexibility and lower the incidence of gout attacks.

By incorporating regular physical activity into your routine can contribute greatly to uric acid regulation and overall well-being.

Chapter 5

Using the Uric Acid Diet to Manage Blood Sugar

Foods that Stabilize Blood Sugar

Certainly! Blood sugar control is essential for overall health, particularly for those with illnesses like diabetes or those who are at risk of getting it. Consuming foods that lower uric acid levels is one dietary factor that has a big impact on blood sugar management. A waste product produced by our body's purine breakdown is uric acid. A uric acid-friendly diet should be followed to promote blood sugar stability because elevated uric acid levels have been linked to an increased risk of insulin resistance and diabetes.

Here are some foods that can reduce uric acid issues while also stabilizing blood sugar:

Low-Purine Foods: To lower uric acid levels, concentrate on eating purine-free foods. Most fruits, vegetables, whole grains, and low-fat dairy products are among them. The best options include berries, tomatoes, carrots, and leafy greens.

Lean Proteins: Choose lean protein sources including fish, tofu, and skinless fowl. Compared to red meat and organ meats, these proteins have lower purine contents, which can result in greater uric acid levels.

Complex Carbohydrates: Instead of refined carbs like white bread and sugary cereals, choose complex carbohydrates like whole grains (such as brown rice, quinoa, and whole wheat bread). Complex carbohydrates help control blood sugar levels by gradually releasing glucose into the system.

Include foods high in fiber in your diet, such as oats, beans, and lentils. Fiber slows down glucose absorption, limiting after-meal rises in blood sugar that happen too quickly.

Healthy Fats: Choose healthy fats from sources like avocados, almonds, seeds, and olive oil. These fats can aid in enhancing insulin sensitivity and lowering inflammation, which is good for maintaining blood sugar levels.

Hydroponics: Water is the best way to stay hydrated. Water intake should be adequate to promote renal function and aid in the removal of extra uric acid from the body.

Moderate Fruit Consumption: Fruits are typically good for you, however, some have more purine than others. The key is moderation, and it's a good idea to speak with a healthcare professional or dietician to find out which fruits are best for your particular requirements.

Limit alcoholic and sweetened beverages: Drinking too much alcohol can alter the way blood sugar is regulated and increase uric acid levels. Drinking too much sugary food or beverages can cause sharp rises in blood sugar levels, so it's better to limit your intake.

Portion Control: Watch your portions to prevent overeating, which can result in weight gain and blood sugar swings.

Consistent Monitoring: Last but not least, it's critical to frequently check your blood sugar levels, especially if you have diabetes or are at risk of developing it. This will assist you in making the essential dietary and lifestyle changes.

It is best to engage with a healthcare professional or registered dietitian who can develop a customized uric acid-friendly and blood sugar-stabilizing meal plan tailored to your unique needs and tastes. Individual responses to food can vary, so it is important to keep this in mind. Additionally, eating a balanced diet is only one part of controlling blood sugar; regular exercise and stress reduction are also crucial for maintaining general health and preventing diabetes.

Meal Preparation for Blood Sugar Management

Particularly for people with diabetes or those trying to avoid blood sugar spikes and crashes, meal preparation is essential for controlling blood sugar levels. A well-planned meal schedule can support sustaining stable blood sugar levels throughout the day. Here is a guide to making Meals to control blood sugar and Regular Blood Sugar Managemen

Balanced meals that are friendly to uric acid Prepare balanced meals with a focus on purine-free ingredients. Effective uric acid level management is made possible by this method.

Purine-Low Carbohydrates: Pick low-purine carbohydrates like whole grains (quinoa, brown rice), as well as low-purine veggies like leafy greens and carrots. These choices give you long-lasting energy without raising your uric acid levels.

Lean proteins with lower purine levels: Include lean protein sources such as fish, tofu, fish without skin, and low-fat dairy products. These proteins contain less purine than red meat and organ meats do.

Fats that are good for uric acid Olive oil, almonds, seeds, and avocados are examples of sources of healthful fats. These fats can enhance uric acid metabolism while enhancing the flavor of your food.

Portion Control: Watch your portion proportions to prevent consuming too many calories, which can cause uric acid to build up.

Limit High-Purine Meals: To help maintain lower uric acid levels, reduce or eliminate high-purine meals including organ meats, shellfish, and some kinds of fish (such as mackerel, and sardines).

Hydrolysis: Water is the best way to stay hydrated. Water intake should be adequate to promote renal function and aid in the body's removal of extra uric acid.

Maintain a regular mealtime plan with snacks and meals spread out equally. Your body can digest uric acid more efficiently with the help of this practice.

Snacks with low purine: Choose low-purine options like fresh fruits, vegetables, and low-fat dairy items if you need snacks in between meals.

Mindful Consumption: Pay attention to when you feel hungry or full on your body. Conscious eating can assist in avoiding consuming too many foods high in purines.

Consult a medical professional: Consult a healthcare physician or a nutritionist who specializes in uric acid management if you have questions about your uric acid levels. They can guide you personally and keep track of your development.

Plan Ahead: To ensure that you have convenient options available, make uric acid-friendly meals and snacks in advance. This may make it simpler for you to stick to your dietary objectives.

Experiment and adapt: Finding the diet plan that best optimizes uric acid levels may take some time because everyone's reaction to food is different. Be ready to adapt as your body provides input.

Keep in mind that controlling your uric acid levels is crucial for avoiding illnesses like gout. The key to reaching and maintaining normal uric acid levels is consistency in your meal preparation and dietary choices, together with appropriate hydration and, if required, medication as prescribed by a healthcare specialist.

Chapter 6

Nutritional Support for Increasing Vitality

Foods to Boost Energy and Vitality

It's crucial to select foods that not only help you achieve your objective of uric acid optimization but also give you prolonged energy and vigor. Regarding uric acid levels, the following foods can assist in increasing vigor and energy:

Whole grains low in purine Oats, quinoa, and other whole grains are great sources of complex carbohydrates. They offer a constant energy release while little influencing uric acid levels.

Leafy greens in addition to being low in purines, vegetables like spinach, kale, and broccoli are also a good source of vitamins and minerals that promote general vitality. They offer a sufficient amount of iron, which is necessary for generating energy.

Low-Fat Dairy Items: Yogurt and milk, two low-fat dairy products, can be included in a diet that increases energy. They are rich in calcium and protein, both of which are essential for bone and muscular health.

Lean Proteins: Choose lean sources of protein, such as skinless poultry, tofu, and legumes. These proteins offer the critical amino acids required for muscle repair and energy maintenance.

Fruits: Numerous fruits, such as berries, citrus fruits, and apples, are rich in vitamins and antioxidants that enhance vigor and general health while being low in purines.

Nuts and Seeds: Almonds, walnuts, and chia seeds are full of fiber, protein, and healthy fats. They benefit heart health and offer a constant supply of energy.

Suitable Fats: Monounsaturated fats, which can enhance general well-being and help sustain energy levels, can be found in avocados and olive oil.

Herbs and seasonings: Include herbs and spices in your diet like cinnamon, ginger, and turmeric. Along with flavoring, they may also be able to reduce inflammation and increase vitality.

Water: Maintaining energy levels and achieving optimal uric acid levels depend on staying hydrated. Fatigue and uric acid removal may both be affected by dehydration.

Green Tea: Antioxidants and a small amount of caffeine in green tea can provide you with a slight energy boost without drastically changing your uric acid levels.

Omega-3 Fatty Acids: Omega-3 fatty acids can be found in fatty fish like salmon, mackerel, and trout. These beneficial fats can promote general vigor and have anti-inflammatory qualities.

Probiotic foods: Fermented foods (such as kimchi and sauerkraut) and yogurt with live cultures help improve gut health, which may increase vigor and energy.

Moderation is Important: Even while some high-purine foods may need to be restricted, it's important to keep in mind that not all high-purine foods should be avoided. A balanced diet may nevertheless include some moderation of purine-rich items like specific meats and seafood.

It takes careful meal planning to strike a balance between energy and vitality with uric acid optimization. Working with a healthcare professional or registered dietitian who can assist you in developing a custom food plan that addresses your unique needs and promotes your general health and vigor while controlling uric acid levels is a smart option.

Rejuvenating Recipes and Foods

Yummy meals and foods that help optimize uric acid levels can also be energizing. Consider the following recipes and foods to help you feel refreshed:

Make a stir-fry with **quinoa and vegetables** by starting with low-purine whole-grain quinoa.
- Pack it full of colorful, low-purine vegetables like carrots, broccoli, and bell peppers.
- Lean chicken or tofu are good sources of protein.
- Season with low-sodium soy sauce or homemade low-purine stir-fry sauce.

A smoothie made of berries

In a blender, add strawberries, blueberries, and raspberries to low-fat yogurt or almond milk.

- Add some spinach to boost the nutrient content without affecting the uric acid levels.
- If desired, add a scoop of low-purine protein powder.

Mediterranean Chickpea Salad: Combine the cucumbers, cherry tomatoes, red onion, parsley, and chickpeas.
 - The dressing consists of olive oil, lemon juice, garlic, and oregano.
 - Sprinkle some feta cheese crumbles on top for flavor.

Omega-3 fatty acids are abundant in **salmon,** a fatty fish.
Try grilling a salmon fillet with asparagus.
- Grilled asparagus is served with a drizzle of olive oil.

 - Taste-test and add herbs, such as dill and lemon zest.

Salad with avocado and spinach - Combine baby spinach, sliced avocado, cherry tomatoes, and thinly sliced red onion. Dress the salad simply with olive oil, balsamic vinegar, and a touch of honey.

Bean and Veggie Soup: To make a hearty soup, use low-purine legumes like lentils, black beans, or navy beans.
- Include a variety of vegetables low in purines, such as kale, celery, and zucchini.
- Season food with herbs and spices to add flavor.

Bell Peppers Stuffed: Stuff bell peppers with quinoa, lean ground turkey, chopped tomatoes, and seasonings.

- The filling should be heated through and the peppers softened before baking.

Vegetable and tofu skewers

- Thread low-purine vegetables (such as mushrooms, bell peppers, and onions) and cubes of tofu onto skewers.
- Grill or bake until barely browned.
- Brush with a marinade of olive oil, garlic, and herbs.

Greek yogurt parfait: Add fresh fruit, honey (in moderation), and a scattering of chopped nuts (such as almonds or walnuts) to Greek yogurt for extra crunch and flavor.

In a bowl, cauliflower rice, a low-purine substitute for regular rice, can be used.

- Add stir-fried low-purine vegetables and grilled chicken or tofu to the top.
- Drizzle on some light teriyaki or sesame sauce.

In order to promote general health and well-being, these energizing dishes use ingredients that are not only uric acid-friendly but also nutrient-rich. Remember to consume these meals in moderation and to drink plenty of water to maintain optimal uric acid levels. If you have any dietary restrictions or medical conditions, seek specialized advice from a healthcare provider or nutritionist.

The Effect of Hydration on Vitality

Hydration plays a key role in uric acid optimization and is essential for maintaining vitality. It is impossible to overstate how important proper hydration is for overall well-being as it affects many bodily processes. An examination of the impact of hydration on vitality concerning uric acid optimization is given below:

Kidney Function and Uric Acid Regulation:
Hydration is crucial to the kidneys' ideal operation. The kidneys' capacity to filter and expel waste products, including uric acid, is supported by an adequate water intake.
- The kidneys can process uric acid effectively when the body is adequately hydrated, which helps to prevent its buildup in the bloodstream.
- Inadequate hydration can result in impaired kidney function, which may help uric acid accumulate and raise the risk of diseases like gout.

Preventing Uric Acid Crystals and Gout Attacks:
Dehydration can make gout, a painful condition
brought on by the crystallization of uric acid in joints,
worse.

- Keeping hydrated can aid in the dissolution of uric
acid crystals and lessen the risk of gout attacks.
Hydration improves joint health and lessens the
crippling pain associated with gout by encouraging
uric acid solubility.

Energy and Vitality: Dehydration frequently results
in fatigue, sluggishness, and diminished physical
and mental function.

- Your body works best when you're properly
hydrated, and you're more likely to feel energized
and healthy.

- Staying hydrated promotes physical stamina,
mental clarity, and general vitality, enabling you to
take part enthusiastically in daily activities.

Cellular Activity and Metabolic Rate:

- Several cellular functions, including those involved in metabolism and energy production, depend on proper hydration.

- Water is necessary for cells to carry out biochemical reactions effectively, ensuring the smooth operation of the body's systems.

- Cells can produce the energy required to preserve vitality and support bodily functions when they are properly hydrated.

Cognitive Capability and Mood

 - Dehydration can affect cognitive function, making it more difficult to focus, remember, and make decisions.

- It may also hurt mood, possibly resulting in irritability and a lack of energy.

- Keeping hydrated is crucial for mental sharpness and emotional stability, which are fundamental components of general vitality.

Circulation and oxygenation:
- Hydration promotes healthy blood circulation, ensuring that nutrients and oxygen are effectively delivered to cells and tissues.
- Blood that is adequately hydrated has less viscosity, which makes it easier for it to move through the cardiovascular system.
- For the production of energy and cellular vitality, adequate oxygen delivery is essential.

Digestion and nutrient absorption are both facilitated by water, which is necessary for both processes.

- Maintaining proper hydration helps the stomach and intestines break down food, which makes it easier for nutrients to be absorbed.
 - To keep your body healthy and vital, it's important to make sure it gets the nutrients it needs.

- Blood that is adequately hydrated has less viscosity, which makes it easier for it to move through the cardiovascular system.
- For the production of energy and cellular vitality, adequate oxygen delivery is essential.

Vittality and uric acid optimization are closely related to hydration. You can support kidney function, lower your risk of uric acid-related problems like gout, increase your energy levels, and improve your general well-being by drinking plenty of water. Regular water consumption is a simple yet effective way to support your goals for uric acid management as well as vitality.

Chapter 7
Adopting a Lifestyle for Uric Acid Optimization

Useful Advice for Prolonged Success

A long-term commitment, adopting a lifestyle for uric acid optimization can significantly enhance your general well-being. Here are some helpful tips for reducing uric acid levels over the long term with a lifestyle change:

Hydration as a Practice: Make it a habit to drink water every day. Maintaining proper hydration supports kidney health and aids in the removal of extra uric acid from the body. Aim for eight glasses of water a day, and make adjustments for your activity level and the environment.

A Balanced Diet as the Foundation: Plan your meals with a Balanced Diet in mind. Consider including whole grains, vegetables, lean proteins, and healthy fats as low-purine foods. For you to keep your uric acid levels at their ideal levels, you must be consistent with your dietary choices.

Mindful Portion Control: To avoid overeating, be aware of portion sizes. Smaller, more frequent, well-balanced meals and snacks support weight control, which is frequently associated with a reduced risk of developing gout.

Lower the intake of sugary and high-fructose foods: Reduce your intake of sugary foods and drinks, particularly those that are high in fructose. These may cause peaks in uric acid. When satisfying your sweet tooth, choose healthier, lower-sugar options.

Select Fruits Low in Fructose: Choose low-fructose fruits like berries, cherries, and citrus fruits when it comes to eating fruit. Compared to high-fructose options, these fruits are less likely to affect uric acid levels.

Moderate Alcohol Intake: If you do consume alcohol, do so sparingly. Particularly beer and alcohol can cause uric acid levels to rise. Alcohol consumption can be significantly improved by limiting or avoiding it.

Regular physical exercise: Regular exercise should be a part of your routine. Maintaining a healthy weight and enhancing insulin sensitivity are all benefits of physical activity. Aim for 150 minutes or more per week of moderate-intensity exercise.

Stress management: Use stress-reduction methods like yoga, deep breathing, or meditation. Finding strategies to manage stress is essential for long-term success because chronic stress can affect uric acid levels.

Routine Inspection: Monitor your blood sugar levels as advised by your healthcare provider if you have diabetes or are at risk. Regular monitoring enables you to change your diet and medication regimen as necessary.

Seek advice from a professional: Cooperate closely with a medical professional or licensed dietitian who focuses on uric acid management.

They can monitor your progress, give you individualized advice, and help you make the necessary changes to your plan.

Adherence to Medication: Carefully follow your healthcare provider's instructions if you are prescribed medication for the management of uric acid or other conditions like diabetes. Your management strategy may be hampered if you miss doses.

Lifestyle Evaluation: Examine your habits for anything that might be causing uric acid problems, like drinking too much alcohol or taking certain medications. With your healthcare provider, discuss any adjustments that are required.

Empowerment and Education: Maintain a working knowledge of uric acid management and associated medical issues. You are better able to make decisions if you are aware of the science behind uric acid and its effects.

Continual Medical Exams: To evaluate your general health and make any necessary modifications to your uric acid management plan, make regular appointments with your healthcare provider.

The Long-Term View: Consider lowering your uric acid as a lifetime commitment to your health. For long-term success, maintaining consistency in your dietary and lifestyle choices is essential.

You can maintain long-term success in controlling uric acid levels and benefit from increased overall well-being by incorporating these lifestyle changes into your daily routine and seeking professional advice when necessary. Remember that everyone reacts differently to lifestyle changes, so persistence and patience are essential on your path to optimal uric acid levels.

Including Uric Acid Optimization in Everyday Activities

Making healthy decisions that easily fit into your routine is possible by incorporating uric acid optimization into your daily activities. How to do it is as follows:

Stay Hydrated Throughout the Day: Develop the habit of always having a reusable water bottle on you.

 - Create reminders on your computer or phone to remind you to regularly consume water.

- Choose hydrating snacks like cucumbers, watermelon, and celery to help you meet your hydration goals.

Plan Balanced Meals: Pay special attention to including uric acid-friendly foods like whole grains, lean proteins, and low-purine vegetables in your meal plans.

 - Prepare meals that are uric acid-optimized in advance to make sure that healthy options are available when you need them.

Mindful Snacking: Keep low-fat yogurt, fresh fruit, raw nuts, and other uric acid-friendly snacks in your bag or at your desk.

 Keep healthier substitutes on hand to replace sugary and purine-rich vending machine snacks.

Move Regularly: Look for ways to work physical activity into your daily schedule; for example, schedule quick home workouts in the morning or evening or take short walks during breaks.

Stress Management: Engage in stress-reduction exercises like progressive muscle relaxation, deep breathing, and meditation.
- Access guided relaxation exercises through smartphone applications or online resources.

Smart Shopping: Make a list of foods that are uric acid-friendly.

- Examine food labels to find items with few added sugars and ingredients high in purines.

Cooking with Care: Test out recipes and cooking techniques that are uric acid-friendly.

- Instead of relying solely on seasonings high in purines, use herbs and spices to enhance flavors.

Social Support: Involve loved ones in your quest to reduce uric acid.

- When going out to eat with loved ones, pick a place with a healthier menu.

Track Your Progress: Track your daily water intake, meals, and physical activity using mobile apps or journals.

- To ensure accountability and guidance, discuss your progress with a dietitian or healthcare professional.

Educate Yourself: Set aside time to learn more about controlling uric acid.

- Keep up with the most recent findings and advice on uric acid optimization.

Create Routine Check-Ins: Schedule regular times throughout the day to reflect on your decisions.
- Examine your diet, hydration, and stress levels and make any necessary adjustments.

Celebrate Small Wins: Congratulate yourself for maintaining uric acid-friendly behaviors.
 - Long-term motivation can be sustained with the aid of positive reinforcement.

Long-Term Commitment: Adopt uric acid optimization as a lifelong endeavor rather than a transient objective.
Recognize that achieving and maintaining optimal uric acid levels requires consistency and slow, steady progress.

You can develop a long-lasting, health-conscious lifestyle that not only improves your uric acid levels but also your general well-being by incorporating uric acid optimization into your daily activities. By incorporating these decisions into your daily life, you can be sure that you're always striving for greater health and vitality.

Overcoming Obstacles and Stalls

It can be difficult to get past roadblocks and stalls in uric acid optimization, but with perseverance and a proactive attitude, you can move closer to your health objectives. Here are some methods to help you get past typical challenges and carry on with reaching your ideal uric acid levels:

Dietary Challenges

Obstacle: You have trouble maintaining a low-purine diet over time.

Solution: For individualized meal planning and advice, speak with a registered dietitian with expertise in uric acid management. For meals that are exciting and satisfying, look for original recipes that are uric acid-friendly.

Cravings and Temptations

Obstacle: It can be difficult to resist cravings for foods high in purines or sugar.

Remedy: To satisfy cravings, keep low-purine snacks on hand, such as low-fat yogurt, fresh fruit, or nuts. To acknowledge cravings without giving in, use mindful eating techniques.

Dehydration

Obstacle: Maintaining proper hydration can be difficult, particularly if you have a busy schedule.

Remedy: Make sure you have daily reminders to drink water. To keep track of your intake, think about using a water-tracking app. For convenience, bring a reusable water bottle with you.

Lack of Exercise

Obstacle: It can be difficult to find the time or the motivation to engage in regular physical activity.

Remedy: Increase your activity level gradually and after a small start. Include brief periods of exercise in your day by walking briefly or using the stairs. Make exercising more enjoyable by finding something you like to do.

The barrier that stress and emotional eating present is that they can influence your dietary decisions.

Remedy: Use stress-reduction methods like yoga, deep breathing, or meditation. Find different ways to handle stress, such as talking to a friend, writing in a journal, or taking up a soothing hobby.

You might encounter instances in which your uric acid levels plateau despite your efforts.
Remedy: Recognize that development is not always a straight line. Continue to adhere to your uric acid optimization plan, and if changes are required, speak with your doctor. Consistency pays benefits over time.

Peer and Social Pressure
This barrier may prevent people from making healthy food and beverage decisions.
Remedy: Tell your loved ones about your dietary preferences and health objectives. When dining out

with friends, look for places with healthier menu options.

Medication Challenges

Obstacle: Side effects or forgetfulness can make it difficult to take your uric acid medication as prescribed.

Remedy: Talk to your healthcare provider about any medication-related concerns. If necessary, they can modify your treatment plan or suggest different medications. To stay on track, set reminders or use pill organizers.

Lack of Motivation

Obstacle: It can be challenging to stay motivated for long-term uric acid management.

Remedy: Establish short-term goals that you can achieve, and treat yourself when you do. To stay motivated and accountable, ask friends, family, or support groups for assistance.

Self-Compassion

Obstacle: Be kind to yourself when you experience failures or times of frustration.

Remedy: Recognize that controlling uric acid levels requires effort and sometimes involves ups and downs. Compassionately treat yourself, and concentrate on moving forward with wise decisions.

Keep in mind that optimizing uric acid levels requires sustained effort, and challenges are common along the way. You can keep moving forward with your health goals and eventually achieve optimal uric acid levels by tackling these difficulties with patience, perseverance, and a proactive mindset. In order to overcome these challenges, speaking with medical professionals or experts in uric acid management can be extremely helpful.

Conclusion

The power of choice and conscious living take center stage in the area of uric acid optimization, where health and vitality converge. It's not just a dietary journey; it's a profound transformation of your health—a path that balances controlling your weight, and blood sugar, and reviving your vitality.

You become the designer of your health destiny as you proceed along this path. You can turn your body into a temple of health by choosing low-purine foods, making drinking water a daily ritual, and planning a menu that honors the harmony of whole grains, lean proteins, and the vibrancy of nature's bounty.

However, this journey goes far beyond what is on your plate. It begs you to put on your running shoes, take in the health benefits of exercise, and learn how to manage your stress so that you can nourish not only your body but also your mind and spirit.

Your regular monitoring of your uric acid levels serves as your compass during this journey and is an essential tool for adjusting your course. It serves as a reminder that maintaining good health is a dynamic, constantly changing endeavor and that your dedication to it is unwavering.

This route provides more than just health; it also provides vitality—a state in which energy flows through your veins, in which you greet each day with vigor, and in which you fully appreciate life's priceless moments.

Keep in mind that you can shape your health, vitality, and future as you travel this path. You are taking charge of your health with each uric acid-friendly meal, each glass of water, each step, and each deep breath.

So, view this journey as a profound gift for yourself rather than a burden. Let it serve as evidence of your fortitude, dedication to improving your health, and unwavering spirit. Accept it with open arms because, by pursuing uric acid optimization, you are not only reclaiming your health but also creating a life that is vibrant, fulfilling, and radiates well-being. The power of choice and conscious living take center stage in the area of uric acid optimization, where health and vitality converge. It's not just a dietary journey; it's a profound transformation of your health—a path that balances controlling your weight, and blood sugar, and reviving your vitality.

You become the designer of your health destiny as you proceed along this path. You can turn your body into a temple of health by choosing low-purine foods, making drinking water a daily ritual, and planning a menu that honors the harmony of whole grains, lean proteins, and the vibrancy of nature's bounty.

However, this journey goes far beyond what is on your plate. It begs you to put on your running shoes, take in the health benefits of exercise, and learn how to manage your stress so that you can nourish not only your body but also your mind and spirit.

Your regular monitoring of your uric acid levels serves as your compass during this journey and is an essential tool for adjusting your course. It serves as a reminder that maintaining good health is a dynamic, constantly changing endeavor and that your dedication to it is unwavering.

This route provides more than just health; it also provides vitality—a state in which energy flows through your veins, in which you greet each day with vigor, and in which you fully appreciate life's priceless moments.

Keep in mind that you can shape your health, vitality, and future as you travel this path. You are taking charge of your health with each uric acid-friendly meal, each glass of water, each step, and each deep breath.

So, view this journey as a profound gift for yourself rather than a burden. Let it serve as evidence of your fortitude, dedication to improving your health, and unwavering spirit. Accept it with open arms because, by pursuing uric acid optimization, you are not only reclaiming your health but also creating a life that is vibrant, fulfilling, and radiates well-being.

Appendices

Glossary of Terms

1. Uric acid, is a naturally occurring waste product created when the body breaks down purines and is frequently present in some diets. Increased blood levels of uric acid can cause conditions like gout.

2. Gout: A painful form of arthritis where uric acid crystallizes in the joints, causing excruciating pain and inflammation.

3. Purines: Natural substances that can be found in foods including red meat, shellfish, and some vegetables. Foods high in purines can make uric acid levels rise.

4. Hyperuricemia: A term used in medicine to describe increased uric acid levels in the blood, which are a risk factor for gout and other medical conditions.

5. Allopurinol: A drug that is frequently recommended to treat gout or hyperuricemia by lowering uric acid levels.

6. Dietary Fiber: Plant-based substances that help with digestion and control blood sugar levels. They can be found in whole grains, fruits, and vegetables.

7. Hydrolysis: Drinking enough water is essential to keeping uric acid levels in check and preventing crystal formation.

8. Low-Purine Diet: A diet that limits or prohibits the consumption of high-purine foods to lower uric acid levels.

9. Inflammation: An immunological reaction that occurs naturally and can be brought on by excessive uric acid levels. It plays a part in diseases like gout.

10. Fructose: This form of sugar, which is present in fruits and added to many processed foods, can raise uric acid levels when consumed in excess.

11. Protein: Animal protein is necessary for physiological function, but taking too much of it might raise uric acid levels. Lean protein sources are suggested.

12. Antioxidants: Compounds that can help lower inflammation and shield cells against deterioration can be found in foods including berries, almonds, and green tea.

13. An alkaline diet seeks to balance the pH levels of the body by focusing on alkaline-forming foods (such as fruits and vegetables).

14. Omega-3 Fatty Acids: Beneficial fats that can support heart health and are present in fish, flaxseeds, and walnuts.

15**. Portion control:** Limiting how much food is eaten to prevent overeating, which can lead to weight gain and high uric acid levels.

16. Metabolism: The body's method of transforming food into energy; maintaining a healthy weight depends on a functioning metabolism.

17. Nutrient Density: Selecting foods that are high in vital nutrients but have few calories.

18. Blood Sugar Control: Blood sugar levels must be managed through diet, exercise, and maybe medication. This is essential for overall health and the prevention of diabetes.

19. Vitality: A condition of general health and vigor that can be fostered by a balanced diet and lifestyle decisions.

20. Moderation: The idea to maintain a balanced diet, all foods should be consumed in moderation, especially those heavy in purines or su

Sample Meal Plans

Keep in mind that these meal plans are only broad suggestions; it is crucial to tailor them to your unique nutritional requirements and tastes. If you have gout or other medical issues, you should also get counsel from a healthcare provider or a trained nutritionist.

Day 1: Low-Purine Meal Plan.
Breakfast: Scrambled egg whites with spinach and tomatoes.
- Whole-wheat toast.
- Fancy strawberry fruit.

Lunch:
- Mixed greens and grilled chicken breast.
- A salad of quinoa with bell peppers, cucumbers, and lemon vinaigrette.

Greek yogurt, honey, and a few almonds make a tasty snack.

Dinner:

- Salmon baked with lemon and dill.
- Steam-cooked asparagus.

Brown rice.

Day 2: Vegetarian menu

Breakfast: oatmeal with sliced bananas and chia seeds.

Green tea.

Lunch:

- Mixed greens on the side and lentil soup.
- A whole grain roll.

Carrot and cucumber sticks with hummus make a good snack.

Dinner:

- Quinoa with grilled portobello mushrooms.
- Roasted Brussels sprouts in garlic and olive oil.

Day 3: the Mediterranean menu.

Breakfast: Have a Greek yogurt parfait with fresh fruit, honey, and chopped walnuts.
- Whole-wheat toast.

Lunch:

- Skewers of grilled vegetables and shrimp.
- Salad Tabbouleh.

Sliced cucumber and cherry tomatoes with a balsamic vinaigrette as a snack.

Dinner:

- Baked cod with spices from the Mediterranean.

- Roasted red pepper and eggplant with herbs and olive oil.

– Couscous.

Day 4: Vegan meal plan

Breakfast: a smoothie made with almond milk, spinach, banana, and a scoop of plant-based protein powder.

Brown rice and chickpea and veggie curry for **lunch.**

Mixed nuts and dried fruits are a good snack.

Dinner:

- Sesame ginger glaze on grilled tofu.

- Steamed carrots and broccoli.

- Quinoa.

Day 5: balanced meal schedule.

Breakfast

- Scrambled eggs with cherry tomatoes, spinach, and other vegetables.

- Whole-wheat toast.

Citrus slices.

Grilled lean beef or turkey burger and a side salad for **lunch.**

Cottage cheese with pineapple chunks makes a good snack.

Dinner:

- Chicken breast baked with garlic and rosemary.

- Steam-cooked green beans.

- Sweet potatoes mashed.

These sample menus offer a selection of choices for a diet that optimizes uric acid levels. Pay attention to drinking lots of water, staying hydrated, and eating in moderation. To assist in controlling uric acid levels and improve general health, seek to maintain a balanced, nutrient-rich diet while minimizing high-purine and high-fructose meals.

Uric Acid-Friendly Recipes

In addition to being delicious, recipes that are uric acid-friendly help you achieve the appropriate uric acid levels. The following mouthwatering recipes can help with uric acid optimization:

1. Chicken on the grill with lemon and herbs
Chicken breasts that are boneless and skinless are among the ingredients.

Orange juice

crude olive oil

- Fresh herbs including oregano, thyme, and rosemary - Garlic cloves, minced

- Conditions:

1. Combine the lemon juice, olive oil, herbs, and garlic to prepare a marinade.

2. Allow the chicken to marinate for at least 30 minutes.

3. Completely grill the meat. Serve with a side of steamed veggies or a salad.

2. Quinoa and veggie stir-fry

The components consist of quinoa and a mixture of veggies (carrots, broccoli, and bell peppers).

 - Tofu or lean chicken strips

- Soy sauce without salt

- Ginger and garlic, minced

- Conditions:

1. Follow the packaging's instructions for cooking the quinoa.

2. Stir-fry the tofu or chicken in a skillet with the ginger and garlic.

3. Add the vegetables and soy sauce. meat until it is soft.

4. Top with cooked quinoa.

3. A berry and spinach salad

The components are fresh spinach leaves and a combination of strawberries, blueberries, and raspberries

- If desired, goat cheese

- Walnuts, chopped

- Balsamic vinaigrette dressing with less sugar

- Conditions:

1. In a bowl, mix spinach and berries.

2. Sprinkle goat cheese crumbles and chopped walnuts over top.

3. Drizzle with balsamic vinaigrette.

4. Mediterranean chickpea salad.

Ingredients: diced cucumber, cherry tomatoes, and red onion; rinsed and drained canned chickpeas; chopped fresh parsley; and sliced and pitted Kalamata olives.

Feta cheese, if desired; dressing made with lemon juice and olive oil.

- Conditions:

1. Combine the chickpeas, parsley, olives, and veggies.

2. After adding the dressing, toss.

3. Sprinkle crumbled feta cheese on top, if preferred.

5. Grilled salmon and asparagus with olive oil:

This dish calls for salmon fillets and asparagus spears.

- Lemon zest and dill (for seasoning)

- **Conditions:**

1. Salmon and asparagus with olive oil.

2. Season with dill and lemon zest.

3. Cook the salmon and asparagus on the grill until the salmon is easily flaked

6. The Greek yogurt parfait.

using the following components: Grecian yogurt

Berry mixture

Almonds and walnuts, diced; honey, used sparingly;

Requirements:

1. Place Greek yogurt, berries, and a honey drizzle in a glass.

2. Add chopped nuts to the top for extra crunch.

These uric acid-friendly recipes offer a delectable approach to support your health goals while enjoying delectable tastes. Remember to modify portion sizes to meet your nutritional needs, remain hydrated, and have fun on your journey to uric acid optimization.